2024 LSAT Reading Comprehension Bible

Dr. Dennis Turco

LSAT

Review have reliably demonstrated the LSAT to be the absolute best indicator of first-year graduate school execution, far superior to undergrad grade-point normal. A fundamental piece of graduate school affirmation, the LSAT is additionally the possibly test that assists imminent regulation understudies with deciding whether graduate school is appropriate for them. Some graduate schools will acknowledge tests other than the LSAT for affirmation. □Nonetheless, understudies who need to expand their opportunities for confirmation and be best ready for graduate school are urged to take the LSAT.

The Graduate School Confirmation Test (LSAT) is the state sanctioned test acknowledged by all graduate schools authorize by the American Bar Affiliation (ABA). While some graduate schools additionally acknowledge elective tests like the GRE, and less significantly the GMAT, the LSAT stays the essential graduate school placement test. It is utilized for different reasons and tests a candidate's capacity to utilize rationale, decisive reasoning and understanding skill.

On the off chance that you intend to take the LSAT, knowing the intricate details of the test, having a definite readiness plan and practicing a solid portion of persistence are significant to getting the score required to have been a cutthroat candidate and procure grants.

Getting major areas of strength for a score is in no way, shape or form the main piece of your application that is important, yet it is a vital one. It likewise fills in for of impartially evaluating your first-year (1L) grades and your probable exhibition inside the class associate.

Graduate schools to a great extent utilize a ringer bend, so contrasting your LSAT score with schools' accounted for midpoints can provide you with a smart thought of how you stack facing the opposition. Numerous candidates give weight to procuring either law office temporary jobs or an ideal GPA, yet all candidates need to truly take the LSAT and their groundwork for the test.

In this article, we unload all that you really want to be familiar with the LSAT, including test expenses and design, how long the test requires and normal LSAT score ranges.

For what reason Would it be advisable for you to Take the LSAT?

Assuming you're considering how to turn into a legal counselor, the initial step is to ensure that you comprehend what legal advisors do and that you have an unmistakable sense that this is a vocation that you need to seek after. Whenever you've shown up at that choice, getting ready for the LSAT is your next significant achievement. Created by the Graduate School Affirmation Gathering (LSAC), the LSAT is the main state sanctioned test that is planned explicitly for graduate school and that is acknowledged by each ABA authorize school.

What Subjects Does the LSAT Cover?

While it's anything but an information or knowledge test, the LSAT takes advantage of the abilities that are generally fundamental for prevailing in graduate school. The test was generally separated into five areas: understanding cognizance, scientific thinking, sensible thinking, composing and a variable segment that is utilized to survey new test questions.

Notwithstanding, following the Coronavirus pandemic, changes were made to the test that permitted candidates to step through the exam at home and in a contracted structure. Through the 2023-24 testing cycle, the test incorporates three various decision segments:

Understanding perception

Logical thinking

Intelligent thinking

A fourth segment is likewise managed, however comprises of test future inquiries and isn't evaluated. Starting in August 2024, the scientific thinking area will be disposed of, and the test will comprise just of the perusing cognizance segment, the unscored segment and an extended coherent thinking segment. This part of the LSAT can be taken from a distance or face to face.

In the wake of finishing these segments, all in all alluded to as the LSAT by a lot of people, first time test takers present a composed reaction which is just directed from a distance, frequently called LSAT Composing. All segments of the distant LSAT and LSAT Composing are delegated to guarantee the test's honesty. While many test takers complete the composing part of the LSAT subsequent to stepping through the exam, the composing part can be finished as long as eight days before the date of the LSAT.

Each part assesses fundamental abilities for imminent regulation understudies, including basic perusing, the capacity to distinguish key realities for a situation or text, insightful thinking and composing with hierarchical construction. These abilities are tried all through the graduate school educational plan and evaluation process. Considering that most graduate school classes are surveyed by a solitary, finish of-semester test, developing these abilities is useful all through graduate school.

LSAT Areas

Understanding Perception

Considering and providing legal counsel major areas of strength for requires abilities. Legitimate specialists should have the option to grasp thick pugnacious and descriptive texts, for example, legal disputes, contracts, choices, proof and lawful codes.

This skill goes outside basically ability to comprehend the text and getting a handle on the topic. Regulation experts should have the option to orchestrate these texts, think about them and apply them practically speaking.

The LSAT's perusing understanding segment involves four arrangements of inquiries, each containing a long section and five to eight related questions. Three of the sets highlight a solitary understanding entry. The fourth set presents two more limited sections that are connected with one another. The test taker should contrast these entries with exhibit their capacity to decide the connection between two texts.

The texts in the perusing cognizance area come from different subjects, including those irrelevant to regulation. Topic might incorporate sociologies, inherent sciences and humanities. The texts are trying because of their thickness and refined jargon.

The inquiries might pose to test takers to decide a text's fundamental thought or reason, recognize express and certain data and dissect a text's association and design.

Logical Thinking

The insightful thinking part of the LSAT is otherwise called "rationale games." This part surveys your capacity to figure out what could or should be valid in light of explicit realities and rules.

This segment presents a bunch of inquiries in light of a specific section and portrays a situation. These inquiries are generally irrelevant to the law. Notwithstanding, the inquiries measure similar abilities you could utilize while breaking down a bunch of guidelines, the particulars of an agreement or current realities of a lawful case.

The LSAT's logical thinking area tests your rational thinking abilities in numerous ways. In this segment, hope to decide the right answer for an issue in light of a bunch of connections; reason with restrictive or on the other hand "in the event that" articulations; perceive when two articulations are intelligently same; furthermore, construe truth in view of realities and rules joined with new theoretical data.

The LSAT's scientific thinking segment is expected to be transitioned away from in August 2024.

Sensible Thinking

Since argumentation is key to providing legal counsel, the capacity to break down, assess, build and discredit contentions is vital. The LSAT's legitimate thinking segment estimates these abilities by evaluating a singular's capability in lawful examination.

Like the other different decision segments, the consistent thinking sections are not really connected with regulation. The contentions in this part come from sources like papers, scholastic distributions and promotions, requiring the test taker to look at, examine and assess contentions tracked down in conventional language.

This part asks test takers to respond to single inquiries about more limited sections containing a contention or a bunch of realities. These inquiries are key to legitimate thinking. They might incorporate perceiving the pieces of a contention and recognizing imperfections, making all around upheld inferences, thinking by relationship or deciding what new proof means for a contention.

After the insightful thinking area is disposed of toward the finish of the 2023-24 testing cycle, the LSAT will incorporate two segments committed to coherent thinking rather than one.

Composing Test

Imminent regulation understudies should have the option to take a position in view of given proof and protect the position consistently recorded as a hard copy. This different, unscored segment of the LSAT estimates a test taker's ability to compose, an expertise that is basic for outcome in graduate school.

The composing piece of the LSAT opens eight days before the numerous decision segment. This segment can be taken on request and is administered utilizing programming introduced on the test taker's PC. Competitors should finish the composing piece of the LSAT to see their score on the different decision segment.

What amount of time Does the LSAT Require?

The LSAT requires something like three hours to finish, in addition to the LSAT Composing area. The various decision piece's four segments are each 35 minutes with a 10-minute break between the second and third segments. Test takers have 35 minutes to finish the composing segment.

There's no time to waste in the LSAT. Each segment accompanies thick understanding material, and there are approximately 25 inquiries for every part. Albeit the test is different decision, wrong inquiries are not meant something negative for you.

The amount Does the LSAT Cost?

Test takers ordinarily should pay the LSAT test charge, LSAC's Qualification Gathering Administration (CAS) expense and the graduate school report expense, among other LSAT-related costs.

Test Charge

Each endeavor at the LSAT costs $222, and LSAC doesn't offer the composing segment as an independent test. In any case, in the event that you are happy with your LSAT composing execution and need to retake the remainder of the test, you might do as such without retaking the composing segment.

Accreditation Gathering Administration Membership (CAS)

ABA-supported graduate schools require LSAT test takers to present their scores utilizing CAS, which improves on the application interaction. It additionally normalizes candidate GPAs and records for grade expansion. A CAS membership at present expenses $200 and stays dynamic for a long time.

Through a solitary record, CAS gives admittance to electronic application handling for all ABA-endorsed graduate schools.

CAS Report Charge

CAS likewise gathers a full report of your necessary records and LSAT scores for each school to which you apply. Every CAS report costs $45. Contingent upon the quantity of schools you apply to this CAS report expense can add hundreds to the expense of your applications.

Discretionary Expenses

The LSAT score review allows you to see your outcomes so you can choose whether to keep or dispose of the score. This see costs $45 whenever bought before your test day and $75 whenever bought subsequently.

You can likewise purchase an authority LSAT score report, which incorporates all LSAT scores procured, including no reportable ones. This score report costs $50.

On the off chance that you would like your LSAT score reevaluated, a score review is accessible for $150.

Schools can see all of your authority LSAT scores while thinking about your application, yet the mind-boggling approach taken by schools is to utilize your most elevated official LSAT score while thinking about your application.

How Is the LSAT Scored?

Finishing the LSAT brings about two scores: a crude score and a scaled score. The crude score is the quantity of right responses you have since wrong responses don't represent a mark against your score. This crude number is then changed over into a scale score going from 120 to 180. Each LSAT is one of a kind, and some have somewhat more or less inquiries than others.

Notwithstanding your score taking on two structures, your scaled score is what graduate schools use while thinking about your application.

For what reason Does the LSAT Matter?

With regards to graduate school confirmations, there is a great deal of conversation about the LSAT's significance. In 2022, the ABA chose to permit graduate schools to be test-discretionary start in 2025. Notwithstanding, this doesn't imply that the LSAT is disappearing. As of May 2023, the association has stopped that cutoff time as it thinks about the necessities and viewpoints of various partners.

Right now, the LSAT is as yet the best indicator of 1L scholarly execution, and keeping in mind that not a fitness test, it is an extraordinary device for candidates to utilize while choosing where to join in. All things considered, the utilization of a chime bend all things considered schools propagates the maxim that at most schools being the hotshot than the minnow at the lower part of the class is better. Class situation stays an element with regards to entry level positions, clerkships and open positions for graduates.

The Graduate School Confirmation Test (LSAT) is a state sanctioned test created by the Graduate School Confirmations Gathering (LSAC) that can be taken face to face at a test site or from a distance. It is intended to anticipate a competitor's true capacity for progress during the primary year of graduate school. The LSAT comprises of five 35-minute areas of various decision inquiries in three different thing types: understanding cognizance, insightful thinking and intelligent thinking. A 35-minute composing test might be stepped through after the examination. LSAC doesn't score the composing test, yet duplicates of the composing tests are shipped off all schools to which a competitor wishes to apply. The LSAT is scored on a scale from 120-180.

The LSAT is offered on different occasions every scholastic year. For onlookers of Saturday time of rest, elective test dates are accessible. Assuming that you are intending to go to graduate school promptly upon graduation, it is prudent to take the LSAT by the late spring going before your senior year. This will permit you to get your scores back so as to partake in all early confirmation/affirmations programs and to be at the front of the application cycle at all schools the accompanying fall. Moreover, in the event that you take the LSAT early, you will have the choice to step through the exam again in a convenient design would it be a good idea for you choose to drop your scores or retake the test later. Later LSAT organizations during your senior year can in any case be practical choices, albeit the later arrival of the scores may fairly adversely affect your nomination at schools that work on more forceful moving affirmation. Less graduate schools will acknowledge scores from the February LSAT organization of that very year of anticipated registration albeit higher scores from this test organization might in any case be useful to candidates on shortlists.

Regulation Administrations reports LSAT scores for a considerable length of time, however some graduate schools won't acknowledge a score that is more established than three years. Thusly, in the event that you anticipate working for some time before applying to graduate school, check the life span of your grades at the particular foundations in which you are intrigued.

You should plan for the test. Planning endeavors ought to zero in the two on getting comfortable with the sorts of inquiries posed and the capacity to foster the endurance to get through the test inside its set time limits. Acquainting yourself with the LSAT right off the bat in your school vocation is really smart, particularly on the off chance that you have a background marked by horrible showing on state sanctioned tests. Pick the sorts of courses that will assist you with fostering the abilities important for a solid exhibition on the LSAT: great perusing understanding abilities, sensible reasoning, and the capacity to basically peruse. Having the option to think rapidly and legitimately will assist colossally on a planned test with preferring the LSAT. While a readiness course might be a decent choice for reading up for the LSAT, it can't supplant a trained routine of self-concentrate too. Preceding paying the cost of a planning course, it is smart to put first in the magnificent and free/reasonable readiness materials accessible through the Graduate School Confirmation Board and particularly the Khan Foundation.

The Graduate School Confirmation Test (LSAT) is a state sanctioned test expected for admission to all graduate schools. Your LSAT score will be a deciding variable in the schools you apply to and demonstrate the probability of acknowledgment. The LSAT is offered four times each year.

The test is an inclination test; scored from 120-180 (with 180 being an ideal score). The LSAT has three principal sorts of areas: understanding appreciation, legitimate thinking (a.k.a., contentions), and insightful thinking (a.k.a., rationale games). The genuine test comprises of five areas (each 35 minutes): one understanding cognizance, two consistent thinking, and one logical thinking, in addition to one exploratory segment (which doesn't combine with your score). Moreover, there is a brief composing segment which is shipped off the graduate schools however doesn't factor into your LSAT score.

There are a wide range of approaches for planning for the LSAT however the one normal recommendation is that you recognize three to a half year of the year that you can give to getting ready for the test. The time and consideration committed to planning for the LSAT will harvest more prominent fulfillment with your score.

General counsel

Take the LSAT in June of the year going before the beginning of graduate school. For current understudies that by and large means June of your lesser year. It is suggested that your prep for the LSAT start in January whether you choose for self-review, get mentoring or take a LSAT predatory class. The objective ought to be to take the test just a single time and score all that can be expected. This prescribed timetable permits you to accept your score in July and start exploring the graduate schools you will apply to in the impending fall. With the heaviness of the LSAT behind you, you can focus on sorting out your application materials, for example, drafting your own assertion and reaching people you wish to have compose letters of suggestion for your benefit.

Neighborhood Test Focuses

The LSAT isn't managed at each test community on all testing dates. Moreover, there is restricted focus accessibility for each test organization. You ought to enlist as soon as could be expected, as your possibilities being allotted to your best option test focus are more noteworthy. In the event that you register on the web, you can check test focus accessibility continuously. On the off chance that you register via mail, and both of your test community choices are full or inaccessible, LSAC will dole out you to a middle as near those habitats as could be expected; in any case, LSAC can't ensure that a middle situated inside a sensible separation from your favored focuses will be accessible. Your LSAT affirmation ticket will mirror the adjustment of test focus. Task to a test place not showed in your LSAT enrollment as well as test date change demand doesn't qualifies you for a full discount or a free test community or test date change.

The Graduate School Affirmation Test (LSAT) is the state administered test expected for admission to regulation school. It is made and regulated by the Graduate school Confirmation Gathering (LSAC). The LSAT is a trial of capacity as opposed to information so it is difficult to remember the data expected to perform well on the test. Practice is fundamental for progress. Beginning August 2023, understudy will have the decision to take the LSAT either face to face at a Parametric testing focus or by means of an on the web, live remote-delegated design. The following is the configuration of the LSAT through the June 2024 LSAT organization:

The LSAT comprises of the accompanying kinds of inquiries:

Understanding Appreciation (one 35-minute numerous decision area)

Insightful Thinking (one 35-minute numerous decision area; known as the rationale games area)

Legitimate Thinking (one 35-minute various decision segments)

Trial Area (one extra 35 moments different decision segment from one of the abovementioned, not scored)

Composing (one 35-minute segment; unscored yet shipped off graduate schools). LSAT Composing is taken independently on-line, on-request You should introduce delegating programming on your home PC and take it in somewhere around one year of your LSAT test date.

What is a decent score?

LSAT scores range from 120 to 180. A decent LSAT score is the one that gets you into your school of decision (and maybe assists you with getting some grant cash too). To decide this, you want to take a gander at the LSAT score ranges acknowledged at that school. All schools report their 25th, 50th and 75th percentile scores. To look into a school's LSAT score range, go to the ABA Standard 509 Reports. Recall while your LSAT score is critical, it isn't the main calculate affirmations.

How would I get ready for the LSAT?

Find out more about the test

Get to know the kinds of inquiries on the LSAT. The best spot to begin is with LSAC.org since LSAC is the producer of the test. For an outline of the test visit About the LSAT. After you have perused the outline, survey the example inquiries with clarifications at LSAC's Sorts of LSAT Questions.

Take a coordinated LSAT practice test

Free practice tests are accessible free of charge from LSAC here. You can likewise step through a coordinated examination for nothing by means of Khan Institute. While numerous understudies are anxious about taking a training LSAT before they have begun planning, it is vital to decide a benchmark score so you can ensure you are improving with training. In the event that you take the training test and do genuinely well, you can focus on specific inquiry types and spotlight on augmenting your score. In the event that you take it and don't score well, don't surrender; you haven't begun to study and practice yet. Utilize your score as inspiration to get everything rolling.

Foster a review plan

Consider how you learn and make an arrangement to plan for the LSAT. Is it true that you are great at using time productively and figure you can make a self-concentrate on time and stick to it? Do you advance best from hearing data, understanding data, composing data or a blend of these?

Self-Study:

Numerous understudies concentrate effectively all alone for the LSAT utilizing planning books (see underneath for a rundown of business merchants that distribute LSAT prep books) and practice tests. Solid time usage abilities and the capacity to gain from perusing and rehearsing are expected for this choice. Verify whether the library (Penn State or nearby) have arrangement books you can utilize or simply survey prior to concluding which books to put resources into for your course of study.

Assuming you pick this choice, begin with the free LSAT prep presented through Khan Institute. Then, at that point, add extra Pretests (past LSAT tests that have been delivered by LSAC). The more practice tests you complete, the less shock questions you will experience on the LSAT. Try to audit the finished tests exhaustively, both the inquiries you misunderstand and the inquiries you addressed accurately. It is critical to see each inquiry and why each answer choice is right or mistaken. Keep on taking coordinated practice tests all through your review to measure your improvement. In the event that you are not advancing, find an elective review technique including a planning course.

Think about joining or making a LSAT concentrate on bunch. Here and there it assists with looking into inquiries with another understudy, especially on the off chance that you can find somebody with qualities that are unique in relation to yours.

Readiness Courses:

The following is an example rundown of a portion of the business LSAT courses accessible. This rundown isn't comprehensive however is intended to assist you with getting everything rolling in exploring business LSAT course choices. Pre-Regulation Prompting embraces or suggests no specific business LSAT course.

Plan LSAT Prep

Kaplan Test Prep

LSATMax

Manhattan Prep

Princeton Survey

Power Score

7Sage

Test Masters

Research the different readiness courses accessible. Most business sellers offer different courses with varying hours and techniques for guidance. On-line courses, either independent or live by means of web based video, are more affordable than in-person classes. Once more, decide how you learn and be straightforward with yourself no time like the present administration abilities. On the off chance that the seller offers a free example seminar on-line, take it to get more familiar with the course. Inquire as to whether the organization has a markdown for Penn State understudies, as many do. Subsequent to investigating as needs be, conclude which course best accommodates your learning style and spending plan, then begin rehearsing!

What Is Custom-based Regulation?

Precedent-based regulation is a collection of unwritten regulations in view of lawful points of reference laid out by the courts. Custom-based regulation impacts the dynamic cycle in surprising situations where the result can't be resolved in view of existing resolutions or composed rules of regulation. The U.S. precedent-based regulation framework developed from an English practice that spread to North America during the seventeenth and eighteenth century frontier period. Custom-based regulation is likewise polished in Australia, Canada, Hong Kong, India, New Zealand, and the Assembled Realm.

Figuring out Custom-based Regulation

A point of reference, known as gaze decisis, is a background marked by legal choices which structure the premise of assessment for future cases. Precedent-based regulation, otherwise called case regulation, depends on definite records of comparable circumstances and rules since there is no authority lawful code that can apply to a current case.

The adjudicator managing a case figures out which points of reference apply to that specific case. The model set by higher courts is restricting on cases attempted in lower courts. This framework advances security and consistency in the U.S. legitimate equity framework. Be that as it may, lower courts can decide to change or digress from points of reference in the event that they are obsolete or on the other hand in the event that the ongoing case is significantly not the same as the point of reference case. Lower courts can likewise decide to upset the point of reference; however, this seldom happens.

Custom-based Regulation versus Common Regulation

Common regulation is an exhaustive, systematized set of legitimate rules made by lawmakers. A common framework obviously characterizes the cases that can be brought to court, the strategies for taking care of cases, and the discipline for an offense. Legal specialists utilize the circumstances in the relevant common code to assess current realities of each case and settle on administrative choices. While common regulation is consistently refreshed, the objective of normalized codes is to make request and lessen one-sided frameworks in which regulations are applied uniquely in contrast to case to case.

Custom-based regulation draws from standardized feelings and understandings from legal specialists and public juries. Like common regulation, the objective of precedent-based regulation is to lay out steady results by applying similar norms of translation. In certain occasions, point of reference relies upon the made to order customs of individual locales. Therefore, components of custom-based regulation might contrast between locale.

2 Custom-based Marriage

A custom-based marriage, otherwise called a non-stately marriage, is a lawful structure that might permit couples to be viewed as hitched without having officially enlisted their association as either a common or strict marriage. While customary regulation isn't normal among the U.S., there are various states that have resolutions or consider precedent-based marriage assuming they meet specific necessities:

Colorado

Iowa

Kansas

Montana

New Hampshire

South Carolina

Texas

Various states, including Alabama, as of late canceled the resolutions considering precedent-based marriage.

3 Unique Contemplations

As judges present the points of reference which apply to a case, they can essentially impact the models that a jury uses to decipher a case. By and large, the practices of precedent-based regulation have prompted unreasonable underestimation or debilitation of specific gatherings. Whether they are obsolete or one-sided, past choices keep on forming future decisions until cultural changes brief a legal body to upset the point of reference.

This framework makes it challenging for minimized gatherings to seek after good decisions until famous idea or common regulation changes the translation of precedent-based regulation. Women's activists in the nineteenth and mid twentieth hundreds of years who battled for ladies' freedoms frequently confronted such hardships. For instance, in Britain, precedent-based regulation as late as the 1970s held that, when couples separated, fathers — as opposed to moms — were qualified for care of the youngsters, a predisposition that as a result kept ladies caught in relationships.

Illustration of Precedent-based Regulation

Occasionally, precedent-based regulation has outfitted the reason for new regulation to be composed. For instance, the U.K. has long had a custom-based regulation offense of "insulting public tolerability." Somewhat recently, the specialists have utilized this old precedent-based regulation to indict another nosy action called up skirting: the act of putting an in the middle of between an individual's legs, without their assent or information, to snap a picture or video of their genitals for sexual delight or to embarrass or trouble.

In February 2019, the U.K. Parliament passed the Voyeurism (Offenses) Act that formally makes up skirting a wrongdoing, deserving of as long as two years in jail and the chance of putting a sentenced person on the sex guilty parties register.

What is a straightforward meaning of customary regulation?

Precedent-based regulation is a group of unwritten regulations in light of lawful points of reference laid out by the courts.

Is customary regulation actually utilized today?

Today the US works under a double arrangement of both normal and common regulation. The courts, for instance, work under customary regulation.

What is an illustration of customary regulation?

The idea of custom-based marriage, which recognizes comparable freedoms as those that have a marriage permit to couples that are not formally hitched in the event that few circumstances are met, is one illustration of precedent-based regulation in real life today.

For what reason is precedent-based regulation significant?

Custom-based regulation puts an accentuation on point of reference while permitting some opportunity for understanding. The worth of a customary regulation framework is that the law can be adjusted to circumstances that were not pondered around then by the governing body.

What is UK custom-based regulation?

US customary regulation begins from middle age Britain, nonetheless, today both the US and UK work under a double arrangement of both normal and common regulation.

What Is the Social Liberties Demonstration of 1964?

The Social Liberties Demonstration of 1964 was milestone regulation that tended to the bias happening in the public arena in the U.S. at that point. Through its 11 titles, it restricted separation and isolation in view of race, religion, normal beginning, and sex in business and in every public spot, like schools, lodgings, eateries, houses of worship, and medical clinics.

The Social Liberties Demonstration of 1964 likewise prompted other social liberties regulations over resulting years.

By the mid-1960s, the social liberties development had acquired public thoughtfulness regarding racial boundaries instruction, public transportation, and utilization of public facilities, like cafés and theaters.

Directly following cruel treatment of serene protestors by the police and the homicides of social equality activists, President John F. Kennedy required a significant social liberties bill in 1963.

His endeavors were delayed in the Senate. After Kennedy's death that year, his replacement, President Lyndon B. Johnson, took up the reason. With the backing of activists like Dr. Martin Luther Ruler, Jr., the bill passed in the House and Senate in 1964.

1 In a long time since the law's section, restrictions against segregation have been extended. This is the very thing that the 1964 regulation incorporates, as well as a glance at resulting social equality regulation.

Understanding the Social Equality Demonstration of 1964

The Social Equality Demonstration of 1964 is broadly viewed as one of the best accomplishments of the social equality development. This memorable government regulation restricted separation based on race, variety, religion, sex, and public beginning.

The law applied to state funded schools, government organizations, businesses, confidential foundations that got administrative assets, and the sky is the limit from there. Segments of the law, called titles, tended to approach access in different areas of society.

2 Title I: Prejudicial Democratic Strategies

Title I denied inconsistent utilization of citizen enlistment prerequisites, for example, education tests.

3 Title II: Integration of Public Facilities

Title II prohibited segregation in view of variety, race, religion, or public beginning in cafés, theaters, lodgings, and inns, as well as any remaining public facilities engaged with highway trade. Exclusive hangouts are absolved.

3 Title III: Integration of Public Property

Title III restricted state and neighborhood legislatures from denying admittance to public property and offices in view of variety, race, religion, or public beginning. It included government authorization of equivalent assurance that was ensured by the Fourteenth Amendment.

3 Title IV: Integration of State funded Schools and Universities

Title IV gave the premise to the integration of state funded schools and universities utilizing the equivalent insurance ensures under the Fourteenth Amendment.

3 Title V: U.S. Commission on Social liberties

Title V accommodated the development of the U.S. Commission on Social liberties that was laid out by the previous Social Equality Demonstration of 1957.

3 Title VI: Segregation by Beneficiaries of Government Monetary Help

Title VI precluded segregation by beneficiaries of administrative monetary help and approved government organizations that dispense the assets to research and end or keep such subsidizing in light of their discoveries.

4 Title VII: Separation in Business

Title VII — one of the most extensive areas of the demonstration — tended to approach business amazing open doors by forbidding segregation based on race, variety, religion, sex, or public beginning by national government managers or confidential area bosses with at least 15 workers. It likewise settled the Equivalent Work Opportunity Commission (EEOC).

5 Title VIII: Casting a ballot Insights

This title trained the Secretary of Business to "lead a study of enlistment and casting a ballot insights catching information connecting with race, variety, and normal beginning."

6 Titles IX-X-XI: Requirement

Title IX worked with the development of social equality cases from state courts to government courts. Title X made the Local Area Relations Administration that would aid debates including separation claims. In addition to other things, Title XI managed the cost of respondents blamed for criminal hatred under the demonstration the right to a preliminary by jury. It likewise set punishments.

7 Extra Social Liberties Regulations during the 1960s

24th Amendment to the Constitution

On January 23, 1964, the US confirmed the 24th Amendment to the Constitution, denying any survey charge in decisions for government authorities. Utilization of survey charges in state races was restricted in 1966 by the U.S. High Court.

8 Casting a ballot Rights Demonstration of 1965

While the Social Liberties Demonstration of 1964 expected all electors to be dealt with similarly, the 1965 Demonstration restricted altogether the utilization of proficiency tests, accommodated government oversight of citizen enrollment in regions where under half of the non-white populace had enlisted to cast a ballot, and approved the U.S. principal legal officer to examine the utilization of survey charges in state and nearby races.

9 Fair Lodging Demonstration of 1968

The milestone Fair Lodging Act was endorsed into regulation by President Johnson seven days after the death of Fire up. Martin Luther Ruler, Jr. It prohibited segregation in view of race, variety, public beginning, sex, or religion in lodging deals, rentals, or financier administrations.

10 Social equality Regulations during the 1970s

The following ten years saw the entry of extra government regulation that extended Americans' social liberties.

Training Revisions Demonstration of 1972

Title IX of the Training Revisions Demonstration of 1972 disallowed segregation based on sex.

11 Restoration Demonstration of 1973

Area 504 of the Restoration Demonstration of 1973 restricted separation based on incapacity.

Branch of Training Association Demonstration of 1979

The Workplace for Social liberties (OCR) was made by the Branch of Schooling Association Demonstration of 1979 to examine affirmed infringement of Title VI of the Social Equality Demonstration of 1964.

14 The impact of the workplace has come and gone with the interest of different official organizations in social equality authorization.

15 Social liberties Regulations, 1980s to the Present

The Social Liberties Law of 1964 went through numerous legitimate difficulties.

16 Among the first was Heart of Atlanta Inn, Inc. v. US.

The inn, which served a highway customer base, had long would not lease rooms to African Americans. The inn proprietor contended that Congress didn't have the authority under the U.S. Constitution to boycott isolation in open facilities.

The High Court decided that the trade provision of the Constitution approved Congress to order this sort of regulation.

17 In 1984, on account of Forest City School v. Ringer, a private, church-partnered, co-instructive foundation sued to stop requirement of the Social liberties Demonstration of 1964 and the U.S. government's solicitation for an affirmation of consistence with Title IX's denial of sex segregation.

The High Court decided that Title IX applied exclusively to the establishment's monetary guide division, which got government reserves, and not to the school in general, which didn't.

18 1988 Social equality Reclamation Act

Directly following the High Court choice in Woods City School V. Chime, Congress passed the 1988 Social equality Rebuilding Act to reestablish expansive establishment wide utilizations of government regulations to separation in training based on race, age, and debilitation in governmentally helped programs.

Americans with Inabilities Demonstration of 1990

The Americans with Handicaps Demonstration of 1990 (ADA) is a social liberties regulation that restricts oppression people with handicaps in every aspect of public life, including position, schools, transportation, and all open and confidential spots that are available to the overall population.

22 In 2008, section of the ADA Corrections Act (ADAAA) extended the number of inhabitants in Americans who could be safeguarded under the law by making changes to the meaning of handicap.

23 Social liberties Demonstration of 1991

Reinforcing prior social equality regulation, the Social Liberties Demonstration of 1991 permitted harms for casualties of purposeful work separation.

24 Late High Court Social Equality Choices

Hitherto in the 21st 100 years, the High Court has gone with four milestone choices that broaden and safeguard the freedoms of the LGTBQ+ people group.

Lawrence v. Texas, 2003

Starting in a police capture of two men in Houston, Texas, that prompted a criminal conviction, this case struck down regulations making same-sex intercourse a wrongdoing.

US v. Windsor, 2013

The court struck down a government regulation that denied advantages to wedded same-sex couples. Edith Windsor and Thea Spyer were hitched in Canada. At the point when Spyer kicked the bucket, passing on her home to Windsor, Windsor was denied a government charge exception for enduring mates.

Obergefell v. Ohio, 2014

The High Court decided that the Constitution ensures a right to same-sex marriage. Fourteen same-sex couples and two men whose equivalent sex accomplices were perished documented suit guaranteeing that denying them the option to wed abused the Fourteenth Amendment.

Bostock v. Clayton Area, Georgia, Height Express Inc. v. Zarda, Harris Memorial Service Homes v. EEOC, 2020

On June 15, 2020, the High Court decided that the social liberties regulation that disallows sex separation applies to segregation in light of sexual direction and orientation personality.